GRANDPARENTS' RIGHTS

Jill Manthorpe and Celia Atherton

British Library Cataloguing in Publication Data

Manthorpe, Jill, 1955
Grandparents' rights.
1. Grandparenthood
I. Title II. Atherton, Celia
III. Age Concern England
306.8'7
ISBN 0-86242-079-2
© Jill Manthorpe 1989
Published by
Age Concern England

Bernard Sunley House
60 Pitcairn Road
Mitcham, Surrey CR4 3LL
and
The Family Rights Group

6–9 Manor Gardens
Holloway Road
London N7 6LA

All rights reserved, no part of this work may be reproduced in any form, by mimeograph or any other means, without permission in writing from the publishers.

Editor Nancy Tuft
Design Eugenie Dodd
Production Joyce O'Shaughnessy
Typeset from disc by Richards Associates
London SW16
Printed by Ebenezer Baylis, Worcester

To FDD, a model grandmother

About the authors

Jill Manthorpe is a graduate of the Universities of York and Hull. She is currently lecturing at the Institute of Nursing Studies at the University of Hull and is also undertaking research for Humberside's Care in the Community Programme. Jill is a former Age Concern press officer and is now serving as a committee member of Age Concern East Riding. Jill Manthorpe is married to a barrister.

Celia Atherton, social worker with the Family Rights Group since 1981, qualified as a social worker in 1976. Before joining FRG she worked as a psychiatric social worker for a number of local authorities. Immediately prior to joining FRG she was a team leader for a busy inner London local authority social services department. Celia has extensive experience of advising and representing grandparents with grandchildren on child protection registers or in care. She also teaches social workers on courses which are designed to encourage the development of good practice in using relatives more positively in helping children in care. She has written on many aspects of families and children in care, including access, child protection procedures and complaints procedures.

Acknowledgements

I would like to thank the individual grandparents who have shared their problems with me. Equally deserving of thanks are the organisations listed who provided me with details of their activities, together with Gillian Douglas (University of Bristol, Faculty of Law) for her information, and Kate Wilson and Dr Andy Alaszewski (University of Hull, Department of Social Policy and Professional Studies), who generously helped with information and comments on drafts of this book. Stella Rhind was a quick and accurate typist while John Dunning, Barrister at Law, and Helen Carr (Bradford Law Centre) assisted with 'technical' legal matters. As always, my children's grandmother was invaluable in providing time and space in our three-generational household.

Jill Manthorpe

Contents

Introduction

Foreword

FAMILY DISCORD *12*

FEARS FOR YOUR GRANDCHILD *16*

COURT HEARINGS *20*

CARE PROCEEDINGS AND FOSTERING *22*

DIVORCE OR WHEN PARENTS PART *38*

WARDSHIP *46*

ADOPTION *48*

CUSTODIANSHIP *55*

IF THE PARENTS DIE *59*

WHEN THE PARENTS ARE NOT MARRIED *62*

BECOMING A STEP-GRANDPARENT *63*

FINANCIAL HELP *65*

WHEN GRANDPARENTS SEPARATE *69*

GREAT-GRANDPARENTHOOD *70*

ACCESS TO CHILDREN ABROAD *72*

SPECIAL CIRCUMSTANCES *73*

SOURCES OF HELP *76*

BIBLIOGRAPHY *84*

Foreword

Future social historians may well decide that there was no more important worldwide change in the twentieth century than the increasing fragmentation of the family. It is strange indeed that more has not been done to shore up families who face so many difficulties today. The parents' time, their most precious gift, has become crowded with new duties and diversions, and even their own children can become pushed out. The more this happens, the more urgent is the need to work out new ways of supporting the family, and to make more use of the old ways.

The oldest way in times of trouble is to rely more on grandparents. One of their most important functions in every known society is their reserve role: to act as substitutes ready to step in when the parents are, for whatever reason, not there. In modern western society they could be crucial, coming from a generation when marriages were more stable.

Grandparents represent stability in an unstable world. But the sad fact is that very often they are not treated with the respect they deserve. They are often not allowed to play their reserve role. This is why this book should be so valuable: it tells grandparents, and those who are on their side, what to do to make themselves effective.

The book gives a wealth of practical advice. It also describes the experiences of grandparents who have faced problems themselves. Grandparents who are going through family troubles will realise, reading this guide, that other people have faced and come through the same difficult times, and they will be able to join up with others who can support and advise them.

Michael Young

Young of Dartington

Sociologist Lord (Michael) Young of Dartington is the founder and director of the Institute of Community Studies which has a long history of research into family relationships and the position of elderly people in our society. Institute reports include: 'Family and Kinship in East London', 'The Family Life of Old People', 'Widows and Their Families', 'Loss and Change' and 'Families at the Centre'.

Introduction

This guide has been written for grandparents facing problems in their relationships with the parents or guardians of their grandchildren. The grandparents may have little or no contact with their grandchildren. Various types of relationships may be involved. The grandchildren may be living in a two-parent family, a step-family or an adopted family; they may be in the care of a local authority or wards of court.

The book explains the legal processes which may be encountered by grandparents and the law as it is in England and Wales. It includes information on self-help groups and the work of helping organisations.

Few professionals receive any training about grandparents' rights. So this book may also be used by people who are approached by grandparents for help or advice. Both Age Concern England and the Family Rights Group believe that grandparents deserve to be seen as more than potential sources of love and help. They should also have their own needs more openly acknowledged.

The new Children Bill, which is passing through Parliament as this book goes to press, contains major reform of legislation as it affects children and their families. The emphasis will be on using local authority provision as a last rather than a first resort in time of trouble. Family relationships will receive a higher profile.

These changes will, however, take some time to be put into practice. Meantime grandparents should be aware that improvements in the law are on the way.

Scotland and Northern Ireland
The legal system is different in Scotland and Northern Ireland so this book only applies to people living in England and Wales. However, many of the organisations listed either operate in these countries or have contacts with similar groups.

In Scotland, the Scottish Child and Family Alliance, 55 Albany Street, Edinburgh EH1 3QY is an advice point to direct people to other help available. For people concerned with children in care, there is the Children's Rights Group, 53, St Vincent's Crescent, Glasgow G3 8NG.

In Northern Ireland, there are two support groups for families of children in care. One is Parents' Aid Northern Ireland, at the same address as the Gingerbread Group (for single parents), 171 University Street, Belfast BT7. The other is Parents in Contact, 16 Sydenham Crescent, Hollywood, Belfast BT4 1TX.

In both countries, the local Councils for Voluntary Service will be in the best position to let you know other groups that have been formed or are in the process of being established.

FAMILY DISCORD

This chapter looks at the problems faced by grandparents who cannot see their grandchildren because of family arguments or rifts.

■ *Ernie and Rose* have one daughter, Dawn aged 28. She is married to Kevin and they have two children. Dawn refuses to have anything to do with her parents. She will not speak to them, returns their letters and will not let them into her home. She stops her children having anything to do with their grandparents. This is very distressing to Ernie and Rose. They feel hurt, rejected and embarrassed. Often they feel very angry with Dawn and her husband. They do not know why she is behaving like this and have no idea what to do.

Can the law help grandparents?

The answer is no. Grandparents do not have any automatic legal rights over their grandchildren. This means they do not have the right to make contact or to keep contact with their grandchildren. The law gives all such rights to the children's parents. If they do not want the children to see their grandparents then this is their right.

Exceptions to this are when parents divorce, separate or one of them dies, or when the child does not live with them. These circumstances are discussed later in the book.

Other relatives, for example, sisters, cousins, great-grandparents, etc., have no rights over the children if the parents have not given up their rights.

Do grandchildren have any rights?

Again the answer is no, though when the children reach the age of 18 they are able to make their own decisions as they are fully adult. In practice many children make their own decisions before this.

Healing the rift

Understanding and resolving family feuds and disputes are some of the hardest things to do. You may find you feel and are very much on your own. The following points may be helpful for you to consider:

- Are there other family members who could help bridge our differences?
- How can we keep contact even though we feel and are discouraged?
- How can we stop ourselves feeling bitter, or angry, or experiencing other emotions which may be damaging to ourselves or other family members?
- How can we still keep our hopes that our family will be re-united?
- How can anyone understand our sadness?

There may be some people who can help you see the situation more objectively and thus react in a more positive way:

- local or national self-help groups (such as the National Association of Grandparents, see page 78)
- a minister of religion
- a long-standing family friend, or other relatives
- a counsellor, such as a member of the National Family Conciliation Service (see page 81), a family therapist (see page 83) or an interested social worker.

Self-help groups

There are a number of groups which may be able to help you or, at the very least, share your problem. The National Association of

Grandparents say:

❝ Everyone in this association, organisers and members alike, have at one time or another experienced the same feelings of sadness, bitterness and frustration which you yourself may be feeling at this moment, and we can assure you that we really do sympathise with your problem. ❞

Some grandparents who have been in this position offer these suggestions:

- 'Keep on sending Christmas and birthday cards – it won't make you feel any worse.'
- 'Try not to get too obsessed by it all, it will make you ill or very boring.'
- 'Don't gossip about your family to anyone and everyone.'
- 'Remember to value your other relatives and your friends.'
- 'Don't let your pride get in the way.'
- 'Find an interest outside the home so it's not an obsession.'

The National Association of Grandparents (NAG), see page 78, have a 'conciliation letter' which can be used by grandparents to send to the parents explaining their sadness about being kept apart from their grandchildren. They suggest you copy out the letter and adapt it to suit your circumstances.

NAG produce another letter which they can send from the Association to a parent who is depriving grandparents of contact with or access to their grandchildren. This letter asks that the parent contacts the grandparents or NAG in the hope of getting some discussion started.

As part of their service to grandparents who have tried to make contact with grandchildren but have not been successful, NAG offer a Certificate of Merit, which is a token of the grandparents' efforts and concern.

Other self-help groups are listed on pages 77–83.

FEARS FOR YOUR GRANDCHILD

This chapter explains what is involved when suspected child neglect or abuse is reported.

What can a grandparent do?

If you are seriously worried about the physical or emotional well-being of any of your grandchildren you should tell the social services department so that matters can be looked into.

You can find out where the local office is by asking at the library, or doctor's, or by looking it up under the name of your local council in the telephone book. You may like to telephone first to make an appointment or you can turn up and ask to see the duty social worker.

Grandparents can have a key role in helping both the individual child and the family. They can be the first people to notice that a child is deeply troubled or the child may turn to them because they love and trust them. Always believe the child and do something. Talk immediately to a health visitor or a teacher or telephone the local social services department.

All the professionals involved will listen to you and they do appreciate how difficult it is to let people outside the family know its secrets.

Sexual abuse of children does happen *within* families of all social classes – more so than with outsiders. And it is only recently many adults who were sexually abused themselves as children have felt able to talk openly about how damaging this experience was.

Occasionally people find it easier or more convenient to go to an independent organisation that employs social workers. The

National Society for the Prevention of Cruelty to Children (NSPCC), the Family Welfare Association or a Family Centre or Family Service Unit are examples of organisations that may have local offices listed in the local telephone directory. However, by far the largest number of social workers work in local authority (council) social services departments and they are under a legal duty to promote the welfare of children.

At the appointment you will be listened to and asked for details. If you want your name to be kept in confidence this will be done. You may like to make a note of the name of the person you see.

It was a relief to talk to someone about my fears. I'd kept my suspicions bottled up for some time but she just listened and let me talk. She said she was pleased I'd come, that I had done the right thing . . . . I did feel better inside.

Remember to ask the social worker what is going to happen and keep in touch if you have information you forgot to mention or matters get worse. Ask the social worker to let you know what is happening.

Removing a child from home

In an emergency, where there is fear that a child is being ill-treated or is in grave danger, social workers have the power to remove them from this danger. To do this they can get an order, called a 'place of safety order', by applying to a magistrate. They can do this either by going to court or to the magistrate's home. Under a place of safety order a child will usually be removed from home and taken to 'a place of safety' such as a children's home, a foster home or a hospital. This can last up to 28 days but in some places the order is usually made for a shorter period. There is no appeal that can be made against this order.

IT IS LIKELY THAT THIS PROCEDURE WILL BE REPLACED UNDER THE CHILDREN BILL BY AN EMERGENCY PROTECTION ORDER WITH THE POSSIBILITY OF PARENTAL CHALLENGE.

How can a grandparent help?

This will probably be a very distressing time for everybody in the family. The parents involved will most likely want to seek legal advice but they may also need to talk over their feelings with someone who is understanding and supporting. You may find it difficult to help your adult son or daughter but the following practical suggestions may help:

- Listen and be prepared to hear the same things again and again.
- Go with the parent to any interviews. Make a note of what is said to help make sure you have both understood what is happening.
- Help with any practical details; baby-sitting with other children, picking them up from school, for example.
- Be prepared for your son or daughter to be angry with you, his or her partner and social workers.
- Remember that social workers have a duty to look after the welfare of the child.

There is more about *your* relationship with the local authority when the grandchild is either under a place of safety order or in care voluntarily (i.e. with the consent of the parents) in the section on Care Proceedings and Fostering on pages 22–37.

The Child Protection Register

Children who are suspected of being injured, abused or neglected may have their names put on a Child Protection Register (or At Risk Register, Non-Accidental Injury Register, or Child Abuse Register). In some areas the records are held by Health Authorities or the NSPCC, but usually the social services department is the official agency with prime responsibility. The register is the responsibility of a Joint Child Abuse Committee composed of senior officials of local social services, health services, the NSPCC and the police.

Other children in the family may have their names put on the Register, even if the initial concern is about one particular child. Their names may be taken off the Register if the case conference decides to do this, or they may stay on until they are eighteen.

The Case Conference

If a child's name is on the Child Protection Register this means the case will be considered at a Child Protection Case Conference. This is a meeting where all or some of the various professionals involved, such as social workers, health visitors, teachers, nursery staff, GPs, the police, NSPCC, meet to discuss what help they can give or what action should be taken.

One of the purposes of the case conference is for these professionals to share all their information about the child. This means that anything you may have told one of them, such as a nurse, for example, may be repeated at the conference, although your anonymity should be respected if you have requested this.

Professionals at the case conference may make various decisions, but strictly speaking, they can only make recommendations to the social services department as the conference has only advisory powers.

Plans will be made for the child at this case conference. This may mean the child continues to stay at home with regular social worker visits and medical examinations. Alternatively, it may be decided to confirm that the child should be removed from the family or that court proceedings should be started.

The case conference will usually decide who will be the professional chiefly involved in working with the child – this person will be the 'key worker'.

The case conference may also make decisions about access – who may see or make contact with the child – so it is advisable as a grandparent for you to let the key worker or one of the professionals know if you want to keep in touch and explain why you think it is important for you and the child.

You can write a statement or letter and ask for it to be read out at the case conference. You may find in your area that it is difficult to go along to the case conference as usually only people from official agencies can attend. However, increasingly, some social services departments do invite parents and often give them a copy of the case conference report if they wish.

It is rare for grandparents to be asked to case conferences unless they are going to be involved in caring for the child and the professionals treat them as part of the team. But you can always ask!

Remember if you want to write a statement or a letter you can get advice from various organisations such as:

- A law centre
- A Citizens Advice Bureau or advice centre
- A solicitor
- The Grandparents' Federation (see page 77).

Individuals such as a family friend, minister of religion, or another relative may help you write a letter or accompany you to a meeting with the social services department.

There should be a review of each child abuse case by the social services department at least every three months. Again, you can use this occasion to let the professionals know of your love and concern for the child, of your desire to keep in contact with the child and your wish to be told what is happening.

COURT HEARINGS

Under new Rules (THE MAGISTRATES' COURT (CHILDREN AND YOUNG PERSONS) RULES 1988), social services departments must now let grandparents know if they are going to take, or have taken a grandchild into care. They must make reasonable efforts to find you.

New rights for grandparents

Grandparents should be informed by the local authority that they intend to start care proceedings and they should let them know the date, time and place of the first court hearing. It may be that they send you an official notice through the post, or that they get in contact with you on a more personal basis. After the first hearing, the court will let you know of any further hearings.

Becoming involved

If the local authority intends to take your grandchild into care you are now able to apply to become involved in the court proceedings. You are then a 'party' to the proceedings. This means you would have the right to be represented in court hearings and to attend. You (or your representative) have the right to ask questions of any witnesses and to give evidence yourself. Also you are able to make representations (i.e. suggestions and proposals) about the issues. As a party to the proceedings you are entitled to see the report of the *guardian ad litem* who acts on behalf of the child, as well as any reports from doctors, teachers, probation officers, etc. You must have had 'substantial involvement' at some time. This means your involvement could have happened several years ago, for example the grandchild could have lived with you for a while when young.

If you could not be said to have had 'substantial involvement' but have maintained an interest in the grandchild you may still be able to become involved in the proceedings. You could be treated by the court as an 'interested person' which means you can attend the court and make representation. However, you will not be a party to the case so will have a more limited role at the court hearing. Nevertheless you should still be able to see the report of the *guardian ad litem* and all the other reports.

If you have not received notice of the court proceedings but do have a 'substantial involvement' you may be able to challenge the court decision. To do this seek professional legal advice.

Unmarried parents

If you are the grandparent of a child whose parents are not married, particularly if you are the parents of the father, you may be known as the 'putative' grandparents. You may find that the social worker does not know who you are or where you live. However, social workers should make enquiries from the child (if old enough), the other parent and, if appropriate, other people involved in the child's care.

You will not be informed by the local authority of their intention to take the grandchildren into care if they do not know about you or if they only treat 'legitimate' grandparents as having automatic rights to receive the notice of the court hearing.

However, you may still be entitled to have your views taken into account if you fall into the category of an 'interested person'. This means you have to have an interest in the child's welfare (current, not past) and the court has to think your representations are likely to be relevant to the case and to the child.

The type of contact or 'interest' that the court will consider may include birthday and Christmas card contact but obviously the court still has to consider how relevant your suggestions are to the child's welfare.

Again, as an interested person, entitled to make representations to the court, you should receive copies of reports sent for use in the court hearing.

CARE PROCEEDINGS AND FOSTERING

This chapter discusses ways in which grandparents can achieve a working relationship with the local authority when a grandchild is 'in care'.

Care Proceedings

Now that the **Children and Young Persons (Amendment) Act 1986** has been implemented, grandparents can apply to become parties in care proceedings when a local authority may be trying to remove children from their parents.

Offering your grandchild a home

If your grandchild has already gone into care, or is about to go into care, then don't delay making your offer of a home if that is what you want to do. You may want to offer a home in the short-term or for the foreseeable future. Waiting for a social worker to come and ask what you can offer can sometimes be misinterpreted as lack of interest on your part.

You may know who the social worker is and live close enough to see him or her to explain what you would like to offer. If you do, make sure that you *also* write a letter making your offer known and asking for it to be carefully and thoroughly looked into. Make it clear that you are interested in discussing this offer with the social workers concerned and that you would want to do so before any final decision was made.

Social services departments have different ways of assessing possible foster parents. If your grandchild is in care then you are, in effect, offering to be his or her foster parent, and your offer ought to be assessed in almost the same way as any other foster parent application. Most non-relatives are offering to foster a succession of unknown children whilst you would be offering to foster a particular child or children from your own family. Some local authorities run groups for possible new foster parents to give them more opportunities to think about whether fostering is really for them. You may feel it valuable to join such a group.

In addition, the social worker, often a specialist social worker from the Adoption and Fostering or Family Finding team, will have a number of assessment meetings with those offering homes. References – personal, medical and police – will need to be taken up too. All this may seem daunting and you will most certainly need to be asked all sorts of personal questions often reaching very far back into your past. It is necessary for the social workers to do this if they are to carry out their responsibilities to the child to make sure that they have made the best choice possible for that child's future. In the same way no social worker should turn down your offer of a home without making such a detailed assessment. This would be another way of failing in their responsibilities to that child.

It is useful, when making this sort of offer, to have discussed it with the child's parents beforehand. It is much better if your proposal can be seen to be one that the parents agree with. However, it will also be important to make it clear to the social workers that if your grandchild is placed with you whilst in the legal care of the local authority or by a court, you would abide by the local authority's or court's decisions in relation to your grandchild.

If the social workers think that you are going to shut the door on them they will be worried about how well they will be able to work with you regarding seeing the parents, where the children go to school and so on.

■ *Brian Sharpe*, aged 4, came into care because his mother felt unable to care for him. Over time she decided that she would never be able to care for him again. His grandmother eventually heard of this and wanted to take over his care. Without fully investigating her offer, the local authority rejected it on the grounds that Brian needed a younger two-parent family which had experience of bringing up children. The grandmother had brought up three children single-handed. She persevered with her wish to

care for her grandson and, some three months later, the local authority agreed to discharge Brian into her care. She welcomed their continued involvement through the next difficult year of settling him into her home. Everyone was satisfied with the outcome but this little boy could have gone to his grandmother much sooner if the social workers had shown an earlier interest in his wider family and had sought more knowledge of it.
(Source: Family Rights Group).

Sometimes social workers, if they have just admitted, or are about to admit, your grandchild to care, may be willing to place your grandchild with you immediately and then make the necessary enquiries and assessments later.

Social workers' reservations

Some social workers welcome offers from grandparents, and other relatives, more readily than others. In some departments the social workers have little experience of placing children with relatives and in others there have been bad experiences. Both these can make social workers anxious about taking up your offer. The sort of reservations a social worker may have are often centred around one or more of the causes cited below.

- The social worker may feel that your grandchild would get caught up in disagreements between different members of the family. The very fact of children going into care can cause anger and hurt amongst family members. There may have been disagreements between different members of the family long before that. If it is true that you don't all get on well together all of the time then don't be afraid to say so. It is quite normal for people who love one another to have arguments, to feel angry, hurt and let down at times. Sometimes we can't sort out our disagreements but decide to put them to one side so that we can get along in other ways.

  Not all families operate in the same way. Some families, because of their traditions and culture, will let their angry feelings show more quickly than will some other, rather more reserved families. They may also, just because they have got it out of their system, get over their anger more quickly than families who don't show their angry feelings but still carry the resentments around years later. What is almost always true is that each family does its very best to protect its young children from the bad effects of those disagreements. Research evidence shows that grandparents fostering their grandchildren who are in care are no different. Research by Jane Rowe (1984) showed that where there was hostility between the grandparents and other relatives, usually the child's parents, that was kept away from the children as much as possible and did not cause additional problems for the grandchildren.

- The social worker may be anxious that by placing your grandchild with you the social services department will be losing control and so will not be able to carry out their responsibilities to the child. In recent years social services departments have become increasingly concerned to have 'control' over children for whom they have some responsibility. This might explain why more children come into care through the courts than before and why more parents who place their children in voluntary care later have their parental rights taken over by the local authority. Research evidence suggests that there is no clear link between local authorities having more 'control' (that is legal control) over children and the local authority making better provision for those children. A DHSS working party that looked at the current research stated:

> ... although the need for greater control is usually justified on the basis of better planning and stability, these studies show that it does not necessarily achieve this. ... Compulsion did not appear to lead to more achievable plans or to greater security for the children – at least in the short-term. What it did achieve ... was immediate 'control' over children, parents or both who were regarded as dangerous and disruptive.

(Packman J., *et al.*, 1986)

However good the plans for a child they can only work out successfully if all the adults involved, and the child if old enough, can work well together. Force won't achieve this but some sort of partnership can. And of course that means you being willing to work co-operatively with the social workers too.

- It is important, if your grandchild is placed with you, that everyone, yourself, the child's parents, the child if old enough and the social worker, is absolutely clear about what is expected of everyone else and what the conditions are of the placement. In the experience of the Family Rights Group, and that of many of the families with whom they have been involved, the best way of doing this is to have a written agreement drawn up between all of you. Each of you signs and has a copy which states what is expected of everyone and what will happen if the agreement succeeds or if it fails. You should also agree when you will review it and make any necessary changes.

If English is not the first language of the grandparent then the social worker should make sure that an interpreter takes part and that the written agreement is in two languages. If anyone involved doesn't read or write very well, then a written agreement is still a good idea because other people – friends or a legal advisor – can read it and explain. They could also be there when the agreement is written up in the first place.

■ The social worker may feel that if your grandchildren's parents haven't made a good job of being parents that is because you didn't bring them up very well. The social worker may then feel that you won't make a very good job of caring for your grandchild either. There are really two different issues here. The first is whether parents fail to do their job well because they didn't have a very good upbringing themselves and the second issue is whether, if you have had difficulties raising one or more children, you will then go on to have difficulty raising another child later in your life. Being a parent is a very difficult job. Most of us try very hard to do that job well and most of us succeed. But for some of us the job is just too hard. Sometimes we know it but find it hard to admit, and sometimes we can admit it. If parents can't or don't do their job very well there may be lots of causes for that:

- they may be living in a strange place and have little or no support
- their own relationship may be bad, leaving them unhappy all the time
- they may have very little money and not be able to manage what they do have very well
- they may be mentally ill
- they may find that they never have quite the patience that you often need with children

- they may have no idea about what children, especially small ones, need.

So their problems will not always be the result of poor upbringing.

In some cases, though, you may believe that you weren't able to give your child, the parent of your grandchild, the upbringing that you would have thought best. If that is the case, don't be afraid to admit it because it doesn't mean that you won't be able to do a good job for your grandchild. You may already have evidence of that because you feel that you brought up some of your other children better. Children vary and so do their parents' circumstances. Life may have been more difficult when one particular child was young; you may have been separated, possibly in different countries, from one child for a long time and found it hard to get on well when you did live together. If you've had trouble with one or more children, it doesn't mean you will have trouble with others.

And as a grandparent you will be that much older, and very possibly that much wiser too. Most of us have made mistakes with our children and know that we would do things differently with other children. Research by Jane Rowe demonstrated that grandparents who have perhaps made mistakes with their own children often go on to care very well indeed for their grandchildren.

Placing a child with grandparents

Sometimes children come to live with their grandparents straight from their parents' homes and the arrangement is made just between family members. Sometimes the parent has gone to the social services department for help and the social worker makes an arrangement for the child to go straight to the grandparent. In both these situations the parents keep their parental rights; the social services department has no legal involvement and you have no legal rights.

The local authority may have started care proceedings in the juvenile court and the court could decide to place the child with you but without taking away the parents' rights. They can do this by making a supervision order with a condition of residence with you. The parents keeps their parental rights; the child cannot be removed from you without the permission of the juvenile court and the local authority must supervise the placement.

If your grandchild is already in the care of the local authority then they can decide to place your grandchild with you. If your grandchild comes to you in this way and is the subject of a care order made in the juvenile court or matrimonial court then the local authority keeps the child's parental rights until the court makes a different decision. This is known as the child staying 'in care'. This could also be the case if your grandchild was in voluntary care although here the parents keep their parental rights but the local authority has the legal responsibility of providing for the child's care. In all these situations your formal legal status in relation to your grandchild would be that of a foster parent (some local authorities would call you a '*de facto* foster parent').

If your grandchild is in care then he or she could be discharged from care when coming to live with you. This can be done immediately by the local authority with the parents' agreement if your grandchild is in voluntary care. If your grandchild is on a care order made in the juvenile or matrimonial court then an application would have to be made to the court by the local authority, parents or child to discharge the order.

If your grandchild is a ward of the High Court then an application would have to be made to the High Court to move your grandchild to you. You, or any other party, can make this application (see page 46). The High Court could keep your grandchild as a ward but give you care and control. It could attach a supervision order to this or it could discharge the wardship order and the parental rights would go back to the parents. The court would be unlikely to take this last course of action if there was still any concern about the child.

If you are given care and control from the High Court then your grandchild cannot be removed without the agreement of the High Court.

If your grandchild comes to you straight from his or her parents or from local authority care you do, at different times, have the right to apply to become the legal custodian of your grandchild or to adopt your grandchild. (See pages 48–54, 55–58.)

Unhappy with the social worker's decisions?

Although it is usually the social worker you will speak to and who will tell you what decision is made, the social worker very often makes this decision with a senior social worker or together with others in a case conference. If you are not happy with the decision then don't be afraid to question it and to ask for it to be reconsidered by more senior persons within the department.

If your appeal is turned down at the first stage then do use the next stage. Don't give up until you have used all the possibilities and if nothing is happening then do push people a bit because someone may be sitting on your appeal.

You may be afraid of being persistent like this and some grandparents have been accused of being too pushy but it is the experience of the Family Rights Group that letting things drift by will rarely be successful. Being a bit pushy may be successful sometimes.

Complaints procedures

Each local authority should have a proper complaints procedure for each of its departments. Information about the social services department should be freely available to you. If you don't know what the complaints procedure is, ask the social worker. If the social worker doesn't know, ask them to find out or write and ask the Director of Social Services yourself. It may be worthwhile to meet with the social worker's immediate superior (usually called a Senior Social Worker or Team Leader) to discuss the problem. Or it may help to meet with the person responsible for the social worker's office (usually called an Area Officer or Team Manager) to see if he or she can resolve the problem.

Most local authority complaints procedures are not very well publicised, but they do exist in some shape or form and they should be used. If you are making a complaint you will usually be asked to write to the Director of Social Services setting out your complaint. Do say in your letter that you would welcome the opportunity to meet the person dealing with the complaint before they make a final decision. Some local authorities also use a special, small panel of elected councillors to deal with serious complaints. Again it may be better if you meet with that panel before they make their final decision.

Help at hand

The Family Rights Group (see page 80) will help families who have children in care or who are involved in child protection procedures. They will give advice about seeking a specialist child care solicitor or, if they are able, they accompany grandparents to meetings with social workers, or appeals panels about access, or write letters on behalf of grandparents.

They cannot give advice on custody cases.

If all else fails

Apart from using the local authority's own complaints or access appeals procedures, there are further ways for you to complain. You can go and see your local councillor, or Chair of the Social Services Committee, at their surgery or write to them. You can also ask your local MP to take up your case. You can find out how to contact them either from your Town Hall or local library.

If all of these means fail then you can make a complaint of maladministration to the Ombudsman (Commissioner for Local Administration). You cannot complain just because you don't like the decision the social services department has made. The Ombudsman, even if he upholds your complaint, cannot change the actual decision that the local authority made. He can only recommend what action the local authority should now take. In order to make a complaint to the Ombudsman you have to show that the way in which the local authority made the decision, or decisions, that you are complaining about, amounts to maladministration and that, as a result, you suffered injustice. You can get more information about how to complain to the Ombudsman from The Commission for Local Administration in England (see page 79).

In the last few years the first cases involving children in care have been taken to the European Court of Human Rights. Cases have been taken both by parents (who won their cases in 1987) and by grandparents (who lost their cases, but this does not mean that other grandparents would not be successful). The case is made on the basis that one or more of the Articles of the European Convention on Human Rights have been broken in relation to yourself. The decisions of the European Court are important because it can mean that the law in this country will be improved as a result. But it is important to remember that taking a case to the European Court may change little for you personally. That is because cases take a long time to be dealt with (the parents' cases took six years) and also because the European Court cannot change the actual decisions in your particular case. If you are interested in taking your case to the European Court you will need expert help. You should be able to get this from a solicitor or by contacting a family support group for children in care, or by contacting Interights (see page 81).

Getting to see your grandchild in care

If your grandchild is in care and you would like to see him or her or would like to keep in touch in any other way then the first thing to do is *ask!*. Don't wait for the social worker to seek you out. Get in touch and explain your interest and say what arrangements you would like to make. The government has issued a Code of Practice on access setting out how social workers should deal with access matters. It is reproduced at the end of the Family Rights Group booklet on access, *Promoting Links: keeping children and families in touch*. This Code makes clear the importance of access by a child in care to his or her wider family.

You may find it easier to write to the social worker asking for access or you may prefer to go to see the social worker personally. Whichever you do, do be sure to explain to the social worker why you think it would be good for your grandchild to see you. Social workers are under a legal duty to make their decisions on the basis of what they believe to be best for the child. They wouldn't be acting legally if they made arrangements just because you would like it. They have to believe that at the very least your access would not be damaging to your grandchild and they have to work to the Code of Practice's guidance that:

' planning will generally be based on the assumption that access will be beneficial to the child unless there are clear indications to the contrary. . . . '

(Source: DHSS, Code of Practice: Access to Children in Care, Paragraph 9)

Continuing links

Sometimes, when you feel very close to people, and even more so when you're feeling unhappy about what's happened to them, it can be difficult to put your feelings and reasons into words and so it could be hard to explain clearly why you want to see your grandchild. You may just feel that you want to see them because they are yours or because they are part of your family. And those, of course, are the very reasons why most of us feel so strongly about our family. They are perfectly good reasons but you may need to explain more to the social worker including why you feel that contact is helpful to the child. Your grandchild is likely to have been seeing you before he or she went into care and it is good for children to keep up as many normal activities as possible after they go into care. That gives them some continuity and of course your relationship with them can be the same whether they live with their parents or someone else.

All that is true, even in those very situations where your grandchild is not allowed to see his or her parents. Research by Jane Rowe found:

' Contact with grandparents was almost always positive. Friction between foster parents and grandparents seemed minimal and children gained a lot. It seemed a great pity that more was not done to promote grandparents' involvement, and it was noteworthy that all eight cases where grandparents stayed in touch after parents dropped out proved to come from just one of the study authorities. It seems unlikely that this could have been mere coincidence. **"**

Sometimes grandparents are reluctant to ask for access in these situations because they are afraid that the child's parents may be against it. It is always better to discuss your hopes with the child's parents whether they are seeing the child or not. If they are not seeing their child they may find it comforting that someone in the family is. If, sadly, they are opposed to your seeing their child that shouldn't really stop you asking the social worker. Except in situations where the child is in voluntary care the final decision is always with the social worker.

When you write to or see the social worker do be sure to explain your willingness to co-operate with them and their plans for your grandchild. They may welcome your approach or they may be slightly anxious about it for the sort of reasons mentioned previously. In addition, the social worker may be worried about too many people visiting the child and so may say that access is for the parents alone. Don't settle for that. Children see lots of people and if there are difficulties they are more likely to be for the social worker in setting up the arrangements than for the child in seeing you. Relatives, such as grandparents, have often been ignored in the past so your request may come as a surprise to the social worker. Don't be rude or aggressive but persist with your request that your grandchild has the chance to spend time with you, just like other grandchildren not in care would. Tell the social worker what sort of involvement you had with your grandchild before he or she went into care.

If the social worker agrees to you seeing your grandchild the arrangements should be confirmed in writing. Do be sure to keep to those arrangements and only make changes if everyone has agreed. If the social worker refuses you access or makes arrangements that you aren't happy with, then ask for the decision to be given in writing. The letter should explain how and why that particular decision was reached. It should also tell you what the local authority's access appeals procedures are (see paragraphs 28 to 31 of the Code of Practice).

Making an appeal

If you are not happy about the social worker's decisions then use the appeals procedure. You should have been told about this by the social worker. If the social worker doesn't know what it is, or won't tell you, then either write and ask the Director of Social Services or ask the Family Rights Group. As you will see from the Code of Practice on access reproduced in the Family Rights Group booklet the procedure should have three stages. First, a senior officer (often the Team Leader or Area Officer) should consider your appeal, second, the Director of Social Services should do so, and finally, if you still can't reach agreement, the elected councillors of the Social Services Committee or a small panel of councillors should consider your appeal.

Sometimes the Director lets the appeal go straight to councillors and at other times you may wish to suggest that the first stage (to the Team Leader or Area Officer) is bypassed. That would most commonly be because you know that they have already been involved in making the decisions that you are appealing against.

You should find out how you can put your point of view to the person/persons dealing with your appeal. You should be able to write to them and it is often better if you can meet them in person too. Anyone who can't write very well should get someone to help. Similarly, anyone who can't write or speak English very well should get an interpreter to help them. The social worker may also be in touch with people who could act as an interpreter. Otherwise they should ask the local Citizens Advice Bureau or Council for Voluntary Service (addresses in telephone book).

It is also worth asking to see the report that the social worker will put forward so that you can comment on it.

When you do write to, or meet with, those considering your appeal, explain why you are unhappy with the social worker's decision and what arrangements for access you would like. It may be that with some further explanation they will feel able to change the decision. It may, for instance, be that your background, traditions or religion are different from the social worker's and he or she didn't understand why you made the request that you did.

Visiting your grandchild

If you do see your grandchild then we know you will want to have as enjoyable a time as possible. And usually that is the way it works out. But sometimes because you are cross with the social worker or because you feel so sorry for your grandchild, you may do things which in the long run aren't helpful. Here are situations to avoid during access visits:

Don't make promises you can't keep   We all want our young relatives to think that things are going to get better and we can be tempted into trying to cheer them up for the moment by a promise of better things to come. But in reality the best gift you can give your grandchild is honesty and your love. Grandparents, whether their grandchildren are in care or not, have little control over them so please don't say you will visit more than you can, or are allowed to, and don't tell your grandchild that he or she will be coming home soon if you have no control over that decision.

Don't say negative things about social workers, foster parents or residential social workers   You may at times feel angry with any of these people but it will never help your grandchild if you tell him or her. It will only confuse your grandchild and make him or her feel torn between you and the others. Adults do disagree and argue but they should not do this in front of the children, and nor should they tell the children later. That can be very hard at times but in the long-run your grandchildren will find it easier and happier to be with you if you don't involve them in your arguments.

Don't bring too many presents   All children love presents and all of us love giving presents to them. We often like doing this even when we can't really afford it. It is so lovely to see our young relatives' eyes light up with anticipation and then to see their frantic excitement at discovering what is in the parcel. And of course giving something pleasurable does make a very clear link with the child. Grandparents separated from their grandchildren in care will feel even more tempted than most to give presents – lots of them. But there are dangers in giving lots of presents. Children love material things and can, if they get too many presents, begin to think of you not as a loving and dependable grandparent but merely as a source of goods. It's not right for a child to think like that, and it's not fair to you, but much worse is the possibility that the social worker will believe that your grandchild only wants to see you for the presents. This may lead the social worker to decide to stop the visits altogether. You may be afraid if you have been giving lots of presents that you can't reduce them. Don't be afraid. In the end your grandchild will love you for yourself and you will find that a lot more satisfying than feeling you have to play Santa Claus every time you visit.

Try to give what you would give your grandchild if he or she were not in care. Probably you would give a present on birthdays and special festivals and nothing or just a small token present on other occasions.

Keeping in touch in other ways

If you can it's a good idea to keep up, or re-make, your relationship with your grandchild in other ways than just by seeing him or her. If you think about keeping up links with others, you don't do it just by seeing them. So if your grandchild is in care, do remember to send birthday cards, and cards at other festivals that your family celebrate. You might also send a postcard if you are on holiday and perhaps the occasional letter too. If you are allowed to phone your grandchild, and feel confident about doing so, then do ring occasionally. All children find telephone calls very special so long as they don't go on too long! And make sure you let your grandchild have new photos of you every now and then. Depending on your grandchild's circumstances he or she might be able to have these where he or she lives and may choose to put the photos into a life-story book.

Many children not able to live with their own families have life-story books. They are like photo-albums but with written memories too so that the child has good background information about what has happened in the past, and his/her origins.

You could also take photos of your grandchild for yourself when you visit. Or if you don't actually see your grandchild, you could ask the social worker to get up-to-date photos for you.

Even if you don't see your grandchild it might be an idea to keep in touch in these ways, so do discuss this with the social worker.

Giving and getting information

If your grandchild goes into care, you may have important information that affects your grandchild's welfare. You may think that the social worker will get this information from others and of course you may be right. In some situations though the social worker may be able to get that information only from you either because you are the only person who has it or because someone else is reluctant to tell the social worker, e.g. that there is a sickle cell condition or epilepsy in the family.

So it's always better to be on the safe side and make sure that the social worker knows about matters you consider to be important. Don't wait for the social worker to come and talk to you. The social worker shouldn't be offended by an approach and if you don't make this contact, the social worker may not know of your existence. Or he or she may interpret your silence as a sign that you aren't sufficiently interested.

The same applies to you being given information by the social worker about how your grandchild is getting on in care or about the plans for your grandchild. If there is something that you want to know then ask. Don't wait to be given information. If you have been quite closely involved in your grandchild's life, or are going to be in the future, then it may be worthwhile for you to take part in his or her statutory reviews. By law these have to be held at least every six months, although they may be held more frequently. The social worker arranges the review and you should ask to take part if you feel you have got something to contribute.

DIVORCE OR WHEN PARENTS PART

This chapter looks at the way you as grandparents can maintain a living relationship with your grandchildren when their parents part. This may be because they get divorced, separate or decide to live apart. This chapter looks at divorce arrangements and some of the ways grandparents have been involved as well as possible complications of access.

> UNDER NEW LEGISLATION IN THE CHILDREN BILL, CUSTODY AND ACCESS IN FAMILY AND MATRIMONIAL PROCEEDINGS ARE LIKELY TO BE REPLACED WITH NEW SECTION 7 ORDERS WHICH COVER RESIDENCE AND CONTACT.

Divorce arrangements

It has been estimated that one in five children will experience the divorce of their parents. When parents get divorced, a court hearing sorts out arrangements for the children. Usually four main areas are discussed in court:

Custody   (legal responsibility for the children)

Care and control   (day-to-day care of the children)

Access   (the arrangements for the parent who no longer lives with the children to carry on seeing them)

Finance   (maintenance money and arrangements about the family home and property).

In most cases arrangements are made between the parents or through their legal representatives, usually solicitors. Sometimes one parent will have custody, sometimes both parents will have custody (joint custody) although the children live with the one parent who has care and control.

Role of the court welfare officer

In some circumstances, the court may appoint a person, known as the court welfare officer, who might interview the parents, talk to the children or see anyone else who may be able to help the court decide what is best for the children. This happens if the parents cannot agree about custody or access. The welfare officer writes a report for the court.

The court welfare officer may come to see the grandparents. You may be visited at home or asked to go for an interview at the welfare officer's place of work. Often a court welfare officer is part of the local team of probation officers but this does not mean there is anything criminal suggested; writing reports for the court is part of the everyday duties of probation officers.

What the welfare officer will be interested in is what is best for the children. He or she may ask you about any arrangements you have worked out between you for caring for the children or about the contact you have with them. For example:

■ **Kath and Tom** were visited at home by the court welfare officer who said she had come to see if they were going to be able to manage looking after 10 year old Luke, while his father was at work. Kath and Tom explained that they often had Luke and his cousins to stay over holidays and weekends and often collected him from school to stay the night. They felt that they were well able to cope physically and really enjoyed Luke's company.

In another case the court welfare officer was not so much concerned with 'inspecting' the arrangements but wanted to check some of the statements given to the court:

■ **Mr and Mrs G** were visited by a welfare officer when their son Mark was applying for more access to his children. He said that he needed more time to take them to visit their grandparents. Mr and Mrs G confirmed this, they said that the children seemed to like visiting them but that their visits were too short to play any games or have a meal, or go to the park.

Sometimes court welfare officers have another role. They may try to encourage the parents to reach agreements about arrangements for access and maintenance, in the hope that this will be better for the children. This is called conciliation; it does not mean they are trying to get the parents back together again. They are trying to sort out arrangements which will work in the years ahead.

Divorce or when parents part

In a few areas there are Family Conciliation Services, either run as voluntary organisations or attached to the probation service or social services departments. Find out if there is one near you by asking at a Citizens Advice Bureau or contacting FIRM (Forum for Initiatives in Reparation and Mediation, see page 80), or the Divorce Conciliation Advisory Service (see page 80).

Third party custody

In some cases, about 400 a year, divorce courts give the custody of the child not to the parents but to someone else, a 'third party'. It is not known how many of these 'third party' arrangements involve grandparents but if *you* are interested in having custody, perhaps because the parents are ill or unable or unwilling to look after the child, you should make your offer known to everyone as soon as possible. In many instances, a pre-hearing agreement will make arrangements quicker and easier.

After a parting

There is no such thing as a happy divorce for grandparents says the *Step-parents' Handbook* from the National Association of Stepfamilies (see page 83). It suggests that among the feelings common to grandparents following the divorce of their child are:

- hurt, pain and anxiety
- shame
- embarrassment
- anger
- helplessness in that they are merely onlookers.

For increasing numbers of people some of these feelings will be intensified because it may be the second time the grandchildren are facing the divorce of one of their parents. Second marriages are twice as likely as first marriages to end in divorce and are more likely to involve children.

Seeing your grandchildren

For most grandparents, seeing their grandchildren after the divorce of the parents will be different in some ways. It may be, for example, that the children do not come to your home so often or that they move away. One set of grandparents describes what can also happen:

‘ Since my daughter got divorced, we have looked after the children every day – taking them to school and fetching them home. We have them during school holidays and half-terms. My daughter works hard and enjoys her career now. She's quite a different girl since her divorce. But it is hard work for us. ’

In some cases, one of the divorced partners goes back to live with the grandparents – either with or without the grandchildren. This can cause some tension once the novelty has worn off. It is probably best to sort out practical details before things get out of hand.

Evidence about grandparents' contact with grandchildren after the parents' divorce is not conclusive. In one study (1981) of children whose parents were divorced, researcher Ann Mitchell found that five years after the divorce, two thirds of the children rarely or never saw one parent. She says that if a child does not see one parent, he or she may well lose touch with that side of the extended family. This compounds the loss for the child.

However, unpublished research carried out by Murch and others and reported by Gillian Douglas and Nigel Lowe of Bristol University's Department of Law, shows that a number of divorced parents said that their children *were* still in touch with grandparents. Of wives with care of the children, 62% said they saw the grandparent frequently (44% in cases of men with care of the children). Only 7% of the wives with care said the amount of contact with grandparents had decreased after the divorce (14% of men).

Despite these figures, there can be a very great depth of unhappiness among grandparents who have been refused access to their grandchildren. They say they feel totally lost, angry, upset, distressed and snubbed. Their distress about the divorce has been made far worse by the loss of their grandchildren:

❛ I felt my ex-daughter-in-law was punishing me in order to get at my son. We'd always got on reasonably well but she suddenly stopped speaking to me and cut all contact. My son had gone to work abroad so I couldn't see the grandchildren when he had them. I felt so wretched, so alone and so shocked. ❜

Grandparents' rights to access

Under the **Guardianship of Minors Act 1971 and Domestic Proceedings and Magistrates Courts Act 1978**, grandparents have the right to apply for access after there has been a custody order made. According to Gillian Douglas and Nigel Lowe (University of Bristol), 100 such orders were made in the Magistrates' Courts in 1984 and 21 orders in the County Courts in 1985. They found that one case a year was the norm for applications in their local Magistrates' Court.

To investigate your own situation you will have to talk to a solicitor, a law centre adviser or Citizens Advice Bureau. As the figures quoted above show, it is unlikely that there will be many professionals who have an amount of experience in this area. You may prefer to see a solicitor who has experience or interest in this part of family law, a member of the Solicitors' Family Law Association, for example. You can consult the Legal Aid list in the local reference library or ask at your local CAB.

The solicitor may well suggest trying to resolve the problem by negotiation or 'give and take'. This is because legal procedures may be slow, complicated and costly.

Going to court

Many grandparents feel that despite the law which allows them access to their grandchildren on the parents' divorce, they are not encouraged to go to the courts. This is because in the experience of many people involved there are likely to be several difficulties.

This might explain why very few access orders are made for grandparents – about 120 each year.

You may get free initial advice from a law centre, Citizens Advice Bureau or a solicitor under the Green Form scheme, and it may be possible to get legal aid. Otherwise you will have to pay for legal representation, letters and telephone calls made by your solicitor. This will be in addition to your own costs – travel to court, loss of earnings, travel to your solicitors, etc.

... The bills do add up. Our bill came to £1,500 and we did not even get a hearing in the High Court as we settled before. Fortunately we are able to pay our solicitor in instalments as he is very understanding.

Nothing will be done quickly, especially if your application for access is disputed by the children's custodial parent.

From our own experience people need to be told to be patient and to try to negotiate – it took us over a year, during which we didn't see our grandchildren at all, it's a very nasty time to go through.

During the time of waiting for court appointments and letters, many people get support from self-help groups of other grandparents who have gone through a similar experience (see pages 77–83).

A shared problem

Shirley Hefferman, Founder of POPETS, the Parents of Parents Eternal Triangle organisation, was herself once parted from her three grand-daughters for nearly three years when their parents separated. She offers the following advice to grandparents in a similar position:

- If you know the grandchildren's address, don't give up writing – even postcards.
- Keep copies of everything you write to everyone concerning the grandchildren.
- Compile a scrapbook of shared memories together.

- If you don't get any acknowledgement of presents you send, perhaps open a savings account for the children.
- Don't give up.

POPETS keeps a confidential register of grandparents who tried to contact separated grandchildren. If grandchildren contact POPETS asking if their grandparents have been in touch, POPETS will forward the grandparents' address, if it receives permission to do so.

Many of the other self-help grandparents' groups listed on pages 77–83 will put grandparents in touch with others in their area so that they can meet or talk on the telephone. All self-help groups have few financial resources, so stamped addressed envelopes are welcome, as well as donations.

One of the aims of the Grandparents' Federation is, for example,

To give support by the formation of local groups of grandparents, by way of advice, friendship and counselling.

For people who are not able to talk about their experiences, most of the self-help groups publish regular newsletters that include comments or case-histories of grandparents who have lost contact with their grandchildren. Reading them may help you see that your difficulties and distress are shared by other people. Some groups are able to reply individually to each enquiry but, as many are small in number, be patient for a reply.

A hollow victory?

One of the difficulties faced by grandparents, and sometimes by the parent who does not have the children living with him or her, is that although access may be awarded by the court it may be virtually unenforceable or not work in practice.

The court was very sympathetic to us but even when you win in law it isn't enforceable. What court is going to lock up the mother of young children because she won't let them see their grandparents?

❝ We were referred to the Family Conciliation and had three meetings – our ex-daughter-in-law only turned up to one. The children weren't present at any – although they should have been – but nothing happened. ❞

Background reading

No-one can predict the outcome of a divorce and how it will affect the grandchildren, their parents or yourselves. It is a worrying time for everyone. Useful publications which you may like to read are:

When Parents Split Up by A K Mitchell published by Macdonald, 1982

Children and Divorce by K Cox and M Deforges published by Stepfamily (see page 83)

Leaflets *Divorce and You* for children and young people, and

Divorce and Your Children for parents, available from The Children's Society (see page 79)

WARDSHIP

This chapter looks at the legal process of wardship which effectively gives the High Court control over a child. It is therefore an extreme step involving time and money and the circumstances are usually highly individual.

NEW LEGISLATION IN THE CHILDREN BILL AIMS TO RESTRICT THE USE OF WARDSHIP BY LOCAL AUTHORITIES.

Although wardship is still a relatively uncommon legal measure, it is being used more to protect children. Wardship proceedings have to be taken to the High Court and, in effect, the court assumes the position of parent to the child. This means the court can make a wide range of orders – among which it can grant or terminate access to grandparents. It can also award care and control of the child to any person who is party to the proceedings, including, of course, grandparents.

As there are still relatively few wardship cases, each case is highly individual. For example, wardships can be used when there are actual or potential dangers, such as kidnapping. Or it can be used to protect a child with drug problems or medical needs. It can also be used to settle disputes between parents or relatives. The court's aim is the protection of the child.

Choosing to start wardship proceedings may well be a long and expensive business for you, though you may feel this is justified by the possible risk to the child of doing nothing. Legal aid may be available to help you with legal costs. In most cases, wardship proceedings are taken by the local authority social services department, but grandparents can initiate or start proceedings; they do not have to have the child living with them to do so. However, if the child is already in care the local authority must give permission for proceedings to be initiated. The Law Commission found that 85% of wardship cases were initiated by the local authority. Grandparents were found to have started proceedings in 61% of those cases that were *not* initiated by the local authority.

■ ***Mrs W*** looked after her grandchildren when their mother went into hospital for a time. When the mother wanted the children back on her return home, Mrs W declined. Mrs W went to court and started wardship proceedings.

In the initial hearing at the court, the case was passed to the court welfare officer to investigate. The Registrar directed that both Mrs W and the mother should be seen with a view to resolving the dispute.

However, the case went on for a long time. It was postponed when Mrs W agreed the children could go back to the mother, but started again when Mrs W felt she was not being allowed to see them enough. The mother was ill again and the children went to stay with Mrs W then they went back to their mother.

Mrs W became ill at the same time as the mother had a further collapse. The children went into care.

The above case illustrates that going to court may not solve anyone's problems. It can be a long process. It can be expensive in time and money.

ADOPTION

This chapter looks at various aspects of adoption and how the grandparents of the child involved may be concerned. It also looks at the rights of grandparents to adopt a grandchild, and suggests alternative arrangements. The ways in which grandparents can keep in contact with a grandchild who is adopted by other people are also considered.

Informal family arrangements

When relatives such as grandparents are involved, it is perfectly legal for a child to be informally placed with them by its parents. This means your grandchild can live with you and no-one apart from the parents (and the Child Benefit section of the DSS office) has to be informed.

Written agreements

In some cases, people who have made an agreement between themselves, within the family, choose to have it written down so that the terms and conditions appear clear for all parties. You can write one for yourselves or go to a solicitor who will listen to your instructions and draft a letter of agreement. You will have to pay for this.

Adoption orders

The only way you can legally adopt a child is through the courts. An adoption order has to be made by a court and it will only do this if it is satisfied that the adoption is in the best interests of the child; the welfare of that child has to be the first consideration. If the parents do not agree the court has the power to rule that an adoption order can be made without their consent.

Although grandparents may know of families where grandchildren were adopted by the grandparents, in practice this is now rare. Adoption is a prime example of a situation where there is a widespread difference between what the law allows and what happens in practice.

Theoretically, if relatives such as grandparents have provided a home for at least 13 weeks for a child then they can apply to adopt the child. The effect of an adoption order is to make the adopters the child's legal parents. The birth or natural parents no longer have any legal relationship with the child.

Even if the idea of adoption is agreed by everyone in the family, the local social services department have to be informed and they will make a written report to the court.

Most social services departments and courts however do not encourage adoption by grandparents. This is because they feel it is confusing for children to change relationships in their families, e.g. grandparents becoming parents.

Nowadays, it is encouraged that adopted children be told as much about their origins and birth parents as they can understand at whatever age they are adopted. It is widely acknowleged that children should not be deceived in any way.

There is an alternative way of having rights to bring up children. This is custodianship (see pages 55–58).

Adoption outside the family

Once children are adopted they lose any legal relationship that they had to members of their natural family. They become the full legal children of their adoptive parents and so it is the new parents who make decisions about who they see or with whom they have contact.

However, some children who are adopted still see members of their natural family – such as grandparents. This can be arranged either in an informal way by agreement, as in the case below, or through the court.

■ *Jamie*, Mrs O'Malley's grandson, was placed in voluntary care by his parents soon after his birth. Jamie's parents felt they just would not be able to cope with him. Mrs O'Malley asked, and was allowed to see Jamie from the beginning. Jamie was placed with foster parents and the original plan was that he should return to his parents' care. However, as time went on it became clear that his parents did not feel able to take on his care and that the social workers would be concerned if they chose to do so.

Jamie's foster parents offered to keep him, and in fact to adopt him. Mrs O'Malley saw Jamie throughout this period and developed a good relationship with his foster parents and his foster brothers and sisters. When Jamie was two and a half he was adopted and it was agreed that he would continue to see his grandmother throughout his childhood. This arrangement has worked well for everybody, not just Jamie. His new adoptive brothers and sisters also enjoy having an extra granny and Jamie's new parents appreciate Jamie, and the other children, having someone extra in their lives.
(Source: Family Rights Group)

You may have been told you cannot have access to your grandchildren because they are going to be adopted. Don't accept that as a reason for not having access.

The points made earlier about letting social workers know of your interest and concern apply here. Let them know, early on, by telephoning and writing that you want to keep up your relationship.

If you have not been awarded access to your grandchildren but do know the adoptive parents' address, then you could write a polite letter to the new parents making known your interest in your grandchildren and your wish to see them. It will be important for the new parents to know that you support the adoption. Unless they feel absolutely certain about this they will never feel secure enough to even think about the possibility of you seeing your grandchildren. If you don't know the address of your grandchildren's new family, ask the local authority, who were involved in the adoption, to forward your letter to the adoptive parents or to their solicitors.

However, the court can make it a condition of the adoption order that a member of the child's natural family should continue to have access to that child. This means the court can order that a grandparent be allowed to visit or see the child. The court will take all the circumstances into account and so you may wish to put your case to the court, either in person or in writing. You could get help with this from a local solicitor or a law centre or you could contact the Family Rights Group, (see page 80) for details of where to go for local specialist legal advice. At this appointment you will need to take along information about the children (names, ages, address, etc.) and to provide details of your relationship with them, e.g. how frequently you have seen them. If you have any copies of letters you have sent to the local authority asking to see the children, or replies, take those along too.

You may be visited by or be asked to go and see a social worker appointed by the court to represent the children in any legal discussion over their future. He or she might be a court welfare officer or a *guardian ad litem*. Although this person is a social worker they are not acting for the local authority applying for any adoption order or freeing for adoption. They represent the children and will listen to their views and may talk to people, like the grandparents, who have detailed knowledge. The guardian's report is then made to the court.

Future contact

If your grandchildren have been adopted in the past or if you have no access, for whatever reason, there are some courses of action you could take now in order to let your grandchildren know at some time in the future of your interest in them and wish to meet up with them.

- You can have a letter attached to your grandchild's first birth certificate. This birth certificate is kept at St Catherine's House, 10 Kingsway, London WC2 and the staff there will attach any letters and photographs you send. When your grandchild is 18 he or she has the right to gain access to his or her original birth certificate and will then see anything attached to it.

- You can also attach this sort of letter to a copy of your Will which can be lodged at Somerset House (see page 61). Even though you may never succeed in contacting your grandchildren during your lifetime, it does give many grandparents a small degree of comfort to know that there is still a possibility of grandchildren knowing of their interest in them at some time in the future.

- There is a voluntary organisation, called NORCAP, which is willing to put separated adopted relatives in touch with their natural families (see page 82). You can write to let them know of your interest in being put in touch with your grandchild if by any chance he or she should ever get in touch with them.

If that should happen in the future then they will help you all make contact. They have many enquiries and now have a computer to store information.

- A number of the self-help groups for grandparents will keep a record of your interest. You cannot guarantee that they will exist when your grandchild reaches the age of 18, neither can you be certain that your grandchild will want to make contact.

Adoption counselling

Every local authority must provide a service for people who have been adopted or who have problems in relation to adoption. This should include counselling help for family members, such as grandparents, who may need to talk about their feelings if they have lost grandchildren; or about problems if they have adopted grandchildren; or who are being asked questions they find difficult to answer on adoption within the family. The local authority social services department may provide this service or it may arrange for a local adoption agency to offer this help.

Although a local authority must now offer such a service **(Sections 1 and 2, Childrens Act, 1975** and **Adoption Act, 1976)**, you may find that in your area it has not yet set up such a service or gives it low priority (Sawbridge, 1988). In London an organisation called the Post-Adoption Centre (see page 83) may be able to help you talk through your feelings.

Adoption in a step-family

You may find that your grandchild is being adopted by a step-parent. This can happen in a number of situations.

■ *Joan's two children* were adopted by their step-father, Alec. Their own father, George, had died three years earlier. Joan knew that George's parents would be worried about this and so she made great efforts to explain to them what was happening before anyone else told them. She explained that no-one could replace them and that they would still be grandparents. She made special efforts to involve them and to keep in touch.

George's parents were welcoming to Alec so that he didn't feel shut out of their relationship with their grandchildren. They didn't make comparisons and referred to him as the children's Daddy. They remembered it would be difficult for him. When Joan and Alec had a baby they treated her as one of their own grandchildren.

Can the grandparent object?

Court decisions vary, sometimes favouring grandparents, sometimes not.

Although in one reported case (Re G (RJ) 1963 1 All ER 20) one of the reasons the court refused permission for a step-mother to adopt was to preserve the paternal grandparents' ties, this is by no means conclusive. In another case (Re F 6th Feb. 1986) the court thought it best to break the family link because of the history of abuse, despite the involvement of the grandparents in the care of the children.

If you do have strong misgivings about the adoption of your grandchildren by a step-parent it is best to try and work out what your doubts are and share them with a sympathetic listener. Another family member may be able to help or if you would rather consult an outsider ask your local minister of religion, someone at the social services department or an advice worker. They may be able to help you separate your own feelings of loss from your concern about the possible harm to the children of losing existing relationships. You may find it easier to then speak to a solicitor if you are clear about your objections.

We take a look at problems in the step-family on page 63.

CUSTODIANSHIP

This chapter explains custodianship, a relatively new arrangement, more flexible than adoption and worth considering for the older child. It gives 'parental rights' over medical treatment and education but does not, like adoption, alter relationships within the family.

If a grandparent or other relative has provided a home for a child for a certain time then he or she is entitled to apply to a court for a custodianship order **(under Part ll of the Children Act, 1975, which came into operation in 1985)**. Various time limits apply. The child has to be already living with you for three months when you apply. If the parent(s) or person who has legal custody does not agree to you becoming the custodian and does not give consent, the child has to have been living with you for at least three years.

You may find that if your grandchild is living with people other than relatives, they may apply for custodianship. For example, foster parents can apply to be custodians if they have given the child a home for at least one year, or three years if the parents do not consent to the application. If the child is in the permanent care of the local authority, then this is the body which needs to give consent if the shorter time periods are to apply.

How does it differ?

Custodianship is not the same as adoption. It gives the successful applicant(s) legal custody of the child, or parental rights. This means rights over matters such as medical treatment, education, religious upbringing, representation, discipline as well as the duty to maintain and protect the child. But the family relationships are not changed. If you apply to be custodians and are successful you are still the grandparents, and the natural or birth parents are still the parents. Unlike adoption, custodianship ends when the child reaches the age of 18 but it can be ended before that on application to the court by the local authority, the custodian or the parent.

To apply for a custodianship order you should go first to a solicitor experienced in family matters or to a social services department office. Some social service departments have written information about custodianship, such as leaflets, which you might like to ask for so you can read about the procedures. A few departments have social workers who specialise in custodianship, but usually you will talk to someone who works with children who are being fostered or adopted.

Once you have made the application, the local authority social services department will prepare a report about you and your family. This confidential report will be shown to the court. They will also contact the child's birth or natural parents to find out their views. Someone will also talk to the child involved to find out the child's views.

What the court has to consider is whether custodianship is best for the child. It has to treat the child's welfare as the first and paramount consideration.

When is it most suitable?

Many social workers feel that custodianship is a good step to take for relatives or foster parents who have been looking after older children for some time. Many such families see the natural or birth parents regularly without any problem, though in some cases custodianship can be used by people who have been looking after a child but fear the parents will suddenly appear, after a long absence, and take the child away.

Some social workers feel that adoption is not appropriate in some cases where children live with relatives. They think such children might feel confused or torn between their birth or natural parents and their adoptive parents.

Custodianship has not been used much because it is a fairly new and unknown procedure. However, knowledge about it is increasing and some social services departments are encouraging people to consider it:

> *Custodianship will be appropriate for children who are well settled with their caretakers, whose placement is intended to be long term, who have a relationship with members of their natural family with whom they wish to maintain contact and who do not need continued support or counselling from a social worker.*

James A and Wilson K 'Social Work and Family Proceedings' 1989

You may find if you have been looking after a grandchild for some time that you are approached by a social worker and asked if you would like to think about custodianship. Some social workers have found that in some cases this can lead to family upset as the child does not know his or her circumstances.

> *The most typical scenario was where grandmother was mum while mother was passed off as an older sister.*

Jane Brooks and Kathleen Batt 'Community Care', 31 March 1988.

Some local authorities pay custodianship allowances to help towards the cost of accommodation and maintenance of the child. Ask the social worker about the practice in your area. The allowances are usually means tested.

If, for example, your grandchild is the subject of a custodianship order, after he or she has been living with another relative or foster parents, then the court can order that you have access to the child. You can apply for access to the child at any time and the court can make an order as it sees fit. However, at any time, the custodians can ask for any access orders to be changed or removed by going back to court.

■ ***Florence Hawley's husband*** had died before she had been able to trace his son from a former marriage with whom he had lost contact some years ago. Very shortly after her husband's death Florence did establish contact with her stepson. She discovered that his own marriage had broken up and after a failed attempt by him to care alone for his two small sons, one had gone to live with a maternal grandmother while the other had gone into care. Florence immediately offered a permanent home to James, her step-grandson in care.

Social workers from the local authority turned down her offer flat, without investigating it at all. When pressed they said James couldn't be placed with her, a) because he didn't know her b) she wasn't a proper relative, and c) she was only making an offer because she was still grieving over her husband's death and wanted to replace him and d) James had disturbed behaviour which she wouldn't be able to cope with.

They were pressed to let Florence's offer be properly and fully assessed by a social worker from the Adoption and Fostering team and to have James and Florence to see a child psychiatrist to see if she could cope with his difficult behaviour. They agreed to do this and after some months both the psychiatrist and a social worker recommended that James be placed with Florence.

James has lived happily with Florence for the last three years. He is now 8 years old and is the subject of a custodianship order to Florence who receives a custodianship allowance from the local authority.

(Source: Family Rights Group.)

IF THE PARENTS DIE

This section covers complications such as disputes, guardianship, access and the implications where wills are concerned.

If only one parent dies

The deceased parent may have appointed a person, such as a grandparent, to be the child's guardian in his or her Will. In this case the guardian will act jointly with the surviving parent. However, many parents' Wills only appoint guardians in the event of both parents dying.

Appointing a guardian

Your grandchild's parents may talk to you about such arrangements when they are making their Wills. They may wonder whether they should have someone younger than you to be the child's guardian, or they may ask you to think carefully about the implications of taking on the task of looking after the children.

If you have been appointed the grandchildren's guardians in the event of their parents' death, you should let them know if later you feel unable to take on the job. For example, your health may have declined. The parents will probably be very pleased you are taking your responsibilities thoughtfully.

Disputes over access

Under the **Guardianship of Minors Act, 1971**, the parents of a parent who has died have the right to apply for access to the relevant child if there is some dispute with the surviving parent. However, Douglas and Lowe from the University of Bristol point out that this excludes the parents of the surviving parent from asking the courts for access if they are in conflict with the surviving parent.

Grandparents in disputes over access should see a solicitor but experience shows that even in these cases there may be difficulty in enforcing access if it is awarded.

When no guardian has been appointed

If a guardian has not been appointed in the parents' Will, then if both parents have died, any interested person, such as a grandparent, can apply to be appointed as the children's guardian. If the children are in care, it may be suggested that you become the children's foster parents instead. Research on foster parents undertaken by Jane Rowe found that many children who were fostered for long periods were with grandparents; however, this option may be less favourably considered by social workers than previously. A recent survey of two local authorities found great variations between the two in their use of grandparents as foster parents for their grandchildren. Some local authorities have a tradition of approving grandparents as foster parents and others think that there should be other people involved or other legal structures used.

In some circumstances, the local authority, which has a duty to take a child under 17 into care if it appears the child has no parent or guardian, may assume parental rights over the child if he or she has no guardian. If a guardian is appointed then the local authority loses these rights.

When there is no legal marriage

In this case only the mother has the power to appoint a guardian in her Will unless the father has custody at the date of his death.

Disputes between guardians

It sometimes happens that joint guardians cannot agree about important matters, such as decisions about education or whether a child should be adopted. It may be that they do not agree over the way the child's money is being spent. Such disputes can be resolved by going to court. The High Court has the additional power to remove any guardian.

Your own Will

You may like to think about what your own Will contains especially in the event of your grandchildren's parents dying before you. What would the grandchildren inherit? Are there articles of sentimental value that you would like to leave to particular grandchildren? What are the tax implications for them? If you have not updated your Will for several years you may like to talk about the possible need to do this with your solicitor.

A Will can be deposited at the Principal Registry of the Family Division at Somerset House, Strand, London WC2R 1LP. Details of the necessary simple procedures can be got from them and it is important if you do this that your executor(s) and solicitor know you have done so.

Along with this document can also be kept a letter or message for a 'long lost' grandchild. On your death, your executor(s) arrange for the opening of the sealed envelope and should try and make contact with the grandchild on your behalf.

WHEN THE PARENTS ARE NOT MARRIED

This makes no difference to your legal relationship to your grandchild unless the parents part. If they live together as a family or have a good relationship of whatever sort then you are as likely to have as good a grandparental relationship as any other grandparent.

You may feel that your grandchildren will suffer as a result of their parents not being married. However, there is nothing you can do about it and it is best not to say anything or interfere. Among your grandchildren's friends there will be many children who live in a variety of family settings so your grandchildren will probably not feel any different.

Your grandchildren, whether their parents are married or not, have equal inheritance rights but you would probably be wise once you have grandchildren, to consider your own circumstances and decide whether you need professional advice.

Access to the child

Under the **Domestic Proceedings and Magistrates' Courts Act, 1978**, the court can grant access to a grandparent, even if the child is 'illegitimate', (Section 14(6)). However, a different situation may pertain depending on the status of the child's parents. It has also been suggested that if a child is not the biological child of one of the marriage partners then only the parents of the biological parent count as grandparents.

However, as the **Family Law Reform Act, 1987** begins to come into force, all parents of a parent of a child will count as grandparents, whatever the marital status of the parents.

BECOMING A STEP-GRANDPARENT

If your child marries or becomes the partner of someone who has children from a previous relationship, you will become a step-grandparent.

Such a relationship will be very much what you make of it. You will have to work out within the family what names you will call each other; what kind of relationship you will have with the children; and how to keep in touch with natural grandparents who may feel they have been displaced by you. Remember, both they and the children may feel confused or anxious about all the changes that are happening in their lives.

Problems in a stepfamily

All of us have problems at some time or other with our children and they with us. However, as the National Stepfamily Association comment:

❛ The stresses of trying to bring up somone else's children – either full-time or part-time – coupled with all the pressures that come from ex-wives and ex-husbands, from access problems, jealousy and guilt – can lead otherwise capable adults to feel totally isolated and total failures. ❜

One of the services offered by *Stepfamily* (National Stepfamily Association) is a telephone counselling service (see page 83). This is a free confidential service, costing only the price of the call, carried out by trained and experienced professionals. It is open to grandparents and all members of stepfamilies, adults or children, so it may be worth letting other family members know about this.

Although this is a relatively new scheme, already several step-grandparents have used this service.

Stepfamily also has a Befriending Scheme, which puts people from the same or nearby areas in touch with each other. This is not a counselling scheme but operates on a purely informal and friendly basis. Befrienders are people often involved in stepfamilies themselves who are ready to talk over the telephone or who perhaps meet for a cup of tea together.

For local groups of *Stepfamily* contact the head office (see page 83) for details. These groups meet regularly in some areas and sometimes arrange special events.

For people who want individual help talking about their family problems or counselling, *Stepfamily* will send their list of specialist Family Therapists covering many areas of the country.

FINANCIAL HELP

This section shows the variety of benefits and the circumstances in which it may be possible to claim financial aid.

Child Benefit and Child Benefit Addition

Child Benefit is a weekly payment to the person looking after a child, Child Benefit Addition is paid to single parents. You may be entitled to claim if you are looking after your grandchild – to do this you fill in a form from your local Department of Social Security (DSS) office. There are special rules for claims which concern children who live in more than one household or who regularly spend part of each week away from home.

Income Support and Housing Benefit

If you receive income support from the DSS or housing benefit from the local authority you may be entitled to extra financial help if your grandchildren come to live with you. Ask at your local office.

Adoption Allowance

This is a means tested payment, based on the boarding out allowance. It is only available in limited circumstances, not to all adoptive parents, and only some local authorities have a scheme.

Boarding Out Payments for children in care

These are payments made to foster parents, that is, *approved* people who have a child placed with them in their home as a member of their family. The payments are not means tested and are not taxable. They are not counted as income for Income Support purposes. You will not get Child Benefit for foster children if you receive a boarding out allowance. The payments vary according to the ages of children and extra payments are available for children with special needs. They are meant to cover expenses.

Custodian's Allowance

This is a weekly payment made to a custodian (see page 57) in some areas. Ask your local authority social services department to consider starting a scheme if there is not one in your area. You might like to join up with other people in similar circumstances to ask for a scheme – contact the Council for Voluntary Service to enquire about local groups of foster parents in your area.

Guardian's Allowance

This is the sum of money paid weekly by the DSS to a person who is looking after a child who is an orphan. You will qualify if you are maintaining the child and either both parents are dead or, if only one parent is dead, the other is untraceable or has been imprisoned for more than five years. If the parents were not married then it is payable on the death of the mother if there is no clear knowledge of the father. If the parents were divorced, it is payable if the surviving parent did not have to maintain or have custody of the child.

It is not taxable, but if you receive income support this will be reduced by the amount of the Guardian's Allowance.

To claim Guardian's Allowance, fill in form BG1 which you can get from a DSS office. You should claim within six months of becoming entitled. If you make a late claim you will only be able to get some arrears (up to six months) if you had 'good cause' for a late claim. If this applies, you should get advice from a CAB, local authority welfare rights worker or law centre on how to establish that you had 'good cause'.

There is more about Guardian's Allowance and the definition of 'good causes' for late claims in the *Rights Guide to Non-Means Tested Social Security Benefits* published by the Child Poverty Action Group (see page 79). Make sure you read the current edition.

Section 1 Payments

Local authorities are under a legal duty **(Section 1 of the Child Care Act, 1980)** to reduce the need to take children into their care or keep them in care by giving advice, guidance or assistance. This assistance can be 'in kind', a bed or high chair, for example; or in cash, for example, money for food in emergencies.

These payments are extremely limited and are sometimes made as loans. Ask at your local social services office.

Visiting your grandchild

If your grandchild is in the care of the local authority and you want to keep contact by visiting, you may be able to get help with your travel costs from your local social services department. They have the power to pay such costs under **Section 26 of the Child Care Act, 1980**, either once or on a regular basis.

If you are refused, you could take your request to a higher level or your local councillor (name and address available from the library or an advice centre). If this is still unsuccessful you may consider making a complaint to the Ombudsman if you think your application was not treated properly.

If your grandchild is not in care you may be able to get help from the Department of Social Security (DSS). If he or she is in hospital or with a parent pending a custody decision you may be able to get a Community Care Grant from the Social Fund. To qualify you would probably be in receipt of Income Support and have savings of less than £500.

If your grandchild is not in these circumstances but you need help with travel costs and receive Income Support, you may be able to borrow money from the DSS, with a budget loan from the Social Fund. This will depend on your local office's priorities and resources.

You do not have to receive Income Support to qualify for what is known as a Crisis Loan, so if there is a desperate emergency (e.g. death, illness or disaster) you may be able to borrow money from the DSS if you cannot borrow money elsewhere. It can only be used for expenses within the UK and again you must not have savings over £500.

You can get more advice on cash help if a child is in care from a booklet *In Care – Money Guide for Families* from the Family Rights Group (see page 80). This costs 50p if a child in your family is in care (£2.00 otherwise).

The Child Poverty Action Group's Welfare Benefits Handbooks are invaluable sources of help about all kinds of benefits and the effects these have on each other. You will find copies at your local Citizens Advice Bureau, advice centre, welfare rights office or social services department.

WHEN GRANDPARENTS SEPARATE

Often when people talk about the consequences of divorce for children they implicitly mean the divorce of a young child's parents. However, about 12,000 people over the age of 60 get divorced each year. Although they do not all have young children to make arrangements for in terms of custody, many grandparents have to work out new ways of relating to their extended family on divorce.

Maintaining contact

It may seem difficult to keep up contact with relatives particularly for men whose wives used to make such social arrangements in the family.

■ *Stan* felt very lonely on his divorce. He did not have his work-mates to talk to now he was retired. He had left his home and so didn't often see neighbours or local acquaintances. Above all he found he missed his grown-up children and the grandchildren who never seemed to call. He felt they kept up the same relationship with his ex-wife but had put him at a distance.

In many families, men have to start to remember special events, like birthdays, when they are on their own. They may have to make an effort to arrange regular contact or things to do. In the case above, Stan found that everyone was pleased when he suggested he might take his grandson fishing on Sundays. Stan always came, no matter what the weather and soon was always expected for Sunday tea. Although he felt embarrassed often meeting his ex-wife at his son's home, he did not let that stop him coming.

GREAT-GRANDPARENTHOOD

With more people living longer, a number of grandparents see their own grandchildren becoming adult and having babies.

At the moment we have little information about the meaning of great-grandparenthood. We know it will vary for individuals because the great-grandparents may be physically or mentally frail, or because they may be living some distance away.

Lack of contact

Sometimes great-grandparents have problems in seeing their great-grandchildren, because of either family discord or family break-up, and the law, as it stands, is of little help. If the children are in the care of the local authority then the great-grandparents, like other relatives, can approach the social services department to ask to see the children. Otherwise there is not yet any experience of cases of great-grandparents being awarded access to great-grandchildren. Like many other relatives you may have to negotiate some compromise rather than sticking to certain principles.

Great-grandparents, however, may suffer from one particular disadvantage. Because of their usually advanced age, other people may think they are 'too old' to be interested. This type of discrimination can take many forms. It may be that someone, meaning well, says 'We won't invite Granny to the birthday party – she'll only find the children too noisy!'. This means older people can find they get left out of some family gatherings. Or it may be that they are unable to do grandparent type things such as giving birthday presents, if they are unable to go to the shops, for example.

Some great-grandparents need help sometimes so that they can form relationships with the youngest members of their families.

- ***Kate*** used to take her baby to visit Elsie, her grandmother who was living in a home. The baby was much admired by everyone and enjoyed all the attention. Elsie loved to see them both, although her memory was failing slightly. Kate said she felt she was giving back some of the love her grandma used to give her when she was a child. She was pleased to have the chance to take photos of her baby and her grandma.

ACCESS TO CHILDREN ABROAD

Sometimes grandparents wish to maintain, or regain, contact with grandchildren who have been taken abroad. There are a number of agencies in existence which can help in such circumstances.

Help available

Families Need Fathers (see page 80) publishes a list of such agencies (price for document pack £3.50 inc p&p). Please specify which country you are concerned with.

One organisation concerned with the law abroad is called Interights (see page 81). You may also be able to get some help from The British Council or International Social Services (see pages 78, 81).

Some people have found it useful to approach their local Member of Parliament in such situations. You can find out the times of your MP's surgery for constituents by asking at the library or an advice centre. It may help if you write a letter beforehand, outlining your problem. All MPs can be contacted at the House of Commons, Westminster, London SW1A 0AA.

If your grandchild is in a country which is in the EEC, then it may be more appropriate to talk to a Member of the European Parliament (MEP). You can find out how to contact your MEP through the library or an advice centre.

SPECIAL CIRCUMSTANCES

This section covers situations where there may be cultural or language differences and/or difficulties. Also included is information on the help available to cope with bereavement.

Problems of making yourself understood

You may be reading this book on behalf of someone who has difficulties in talking to people in official positions. This may be because he or she does not speak English fluently, or has learning difficulties or problems listening or talking to people.

It is important that people with these difficulties can both explain their problems and also understand what their advisors are saying or suggesting they do. They may need interpreters to help at interviews and with translating letters or forms.

An interpreter should also be able to explain particular cultural arrangements or patterns of child-rearing that are the custom in some communities or religions. If no-one explains these to a helping agency then the grandparents' representative will be unable to explain or answer questions.

Language interpreters may be found through the local Council for Racial Equality or the local social services department or court may be able to arrange one. However, it may be wise to arrange to talk with an interpreter before any court hearing to make sure he or she fully understands a particular case.

A grandchild from a different culture or race

Your children may choose to adopt a child from another race or ethnic group. One of your children may marry someone from a different race. Naturally they will want your support and encouragment. In many ways if there has been an adoption the situation is like that of any grandparents who are becoming adoptive or step-grandparents.

You may like to remember that some step-grandparents say that it is sometimes difficult to get over two feelings. The first is that many grandparents tend to seek something of themselves in their grandchildren:

❛ No matter how successful the stepfamily is, nothing will ever make the stepchildren or stepgrandchildren your 'own'. ❜
(Erica De'Ath and Linda Parry Jones *One Step at a Time – Grandparents and Stepgrandparents*)

The other is that some grandparents place great importance on shared family history and so feel a child who does not share a blood tie does not keep up this traditional image. The authors above suggest:

❛ ... there is no reason why some family history can't be learned and shared through photos and celebration of family events. ❜

It is likely that there will be local groups in your area of families who have adopted children or who have mixed race children. Often these meet for a mixture of social events and educational or cultural get-togethers. One example is Harmony (see page 81).

For details of local groups contact the local Community Relations Council.

❛ We have an adopted grand-daughter who is Afro-caribbean. We tried to learn a bit about the island where one of her natural parents came from – it's quite interesting to point Jamaican things out to her. We also read her stories which sometimes have West Indian themes or pictures. One thing we learned about was how to do her hair as she wanted. We are lucky to have her in our family. ❜

If your grandchild dies

The experience of losing a child or a baby in a family can be devastating for some people. Organisations exist that help people who have been bereaved – some are specially for relations who have lost children in particular ways such as through violence or 'cot deaths'.

Compassionate Friends (see page 79) is one such organisation offering mutual friendship and support for relatives following the death of a child of any age. Cruse (see page 79) will put you in touch with a local bereavement group and you might find their leaflets helpful to read. They offer advice and support for all forms of bereavement.

You may find it helpful to talk to someone such as a minister of religion or a social worker or to join other groups of families who meet together through a hospice, a hospital or other voluntary organisation.

SOURCES OF HELP

Support groups

Bringing up a child on your own can be difficult but in many places there are local groups of lone parents or people in similar positions who meet together for friendship, information, advice and company. The largest of these self-help associations is Gingerbread (see page 81), but you may be able to find out about other local groups from a health visitor or Council for Voluntary Service. Such groups are not simply for families with young children; they may be involved in activities such as holiday play-schemes or child-care arrangements for older children.

Law Centres

In some areas, a law centre may be able to give advice on family matters. Their staff may give simple advice, represent you at a court hearing, write letters on your behalf or accompany you to interviews. Not all centres are specialists in the area of family law so they may suggest which local solicitors are most experienced, sympathetic or knowledgeable.

Don't forget to take letters or correspondence you have to interviews and appointments. You might like to take photocopies in case papers get lost.

You can find out if there is a local law centre in your area by asking at the Citizens Advice Bureau or Library.

Local Government Ombudsman

The Ombudsman is the person to whom you can ultimately complain about maladministration within a local authority.

An example of this is a case reported in *Community Care* (21.1.88) in which the grandparents of a child who was made a ward of court and placed for adoption complained that their wish to keep in contact with her was ignored. The Ombudsman did not uphold this particular case but said the social workers should have agreed to meet the grandparents and dealt 'more sympathetically' with them.

See page 29 for more information on complaints procedures and page 30 on making a complaint to the Ombudsman.

Grandparents' Groups

These self-help groups set up by grandparents are often run by a small number of committed people so they will appreciate help with postage. At times they may be under pressure so do not expect an immediate reply.

- **Children Need Grandparents**
  2 Surrey Way, Laindon, West Basildon, Essex SS15 6PS
  Small organisation offering support and advice to grandparents separated from their grandchildren; offers an opportunity for grandparents to share their feelings and can explain the difficulties of going to court in order to gain access.

- **Grandparents' Federation**
  78 Cook's Spinney, Harlow, Essex CM20 3BL
  Tel: 0279 451251
  Organisation for grandparents with young relatives *in care*; it offers advice and support through letters and puts people in touch with others in similar circumstances in their locality: publishes a newsletter 'Grandparents' Times'.
  The Grandparents' Federation refer people for specific legal advice to the Family Rights Group.

- **National Association of Grandparents**
  8 Kirkley Drive, Ashington, Northumbria NE63 9RD
  Offers advice and support, and also campaigns for better access to grandchildren involved in custody or care proceedings; a quarterly newsletter for members and a friendship club for grandparents separated from their grandchildren for whatever reason. Contacts in many areas (including Scotland). Please send SAE when writing. Membership £1.00.

  NAG publish a conciliation letter that may be adapted for use by grandparents separated from their grandchildren; will send a mediating letter to parents if this is thought advisable.

- **POPETS (Parents of Parents Eternal Triangle)**
  15 Calder Close, Higher Compton, Plymouth PL3 6NT
  Tel: 0752 77036
  Grandparents' rights group started in 1984; campaigns for access to grandchildren to be an automatic right of grandparents in times of parental break-up; gives advice to grandparents on how to stay in touch with their grandchildren and keeps a register of grandparents who have been kept apart from their grandchildren so that in later years the grandchildren may be able to trace their grandparents or at least know of their concern. Publishes members' newsletter.

Other Helping Organisations

- **The British Council**
  10 Spring Gardens, London SW1A 2BN
  Tel: 01-930 8466
  May be able to trace children who are British Nationals by contacting schools in the relevant country.

- **Childaid**
  3 Church Street, Heywood, Lancashire OL10 1LW
  A locally based group set up to help children who have been abused, physically or emotionally; members offer support and campaign for legal changes; particularly concerned about grandparents' access to children in care.

- **Child Poverty Action Group and Citizens Rights Office**
  4th Floor, 1–5 Bath Street, London EC1V 9PY
  Tel: 01-253 3406
  If you cannot get local advice about benefits or you have a very complicated legal problem about your benefits, CPAG may be able to help you. It also publishes two 'National Welfare Benefits Handbooks' which are invaluable sources of help. Make sure you consult the current edition.

- **Children's Legal Centre**
  20 Compton Terrace, London N1
  Tel: 01-359 6251
  Gives advice regarding children in care and is a pressure group for children's rights.

- **The Children's Society**
  Edward Rudolf House, Margery Street, London WC1X 0JL
  Tel: 01-837 4299
  Publishes the leaflets *Divorce and You* (for children and young people) and *Divorce and Your Children* (for parents). Offers a range of support for families, including two conciliation services.

- **Commission for Local Administration in England**
  21 Queen Anne's Gate, London SW1H 9BU
  Tel: 01-222 5622
  Free booklet available on how to complain to the Ombudsman for Local Government in cases of maladministration.

- **Compassionate Friends**
  6 Denmark Street, Bristol BS1 5DQ
  Offers mutual friendship and support for relatives following the death of a child of any age.

- **Cruse – Bereavement Care**
  126 Sheen Road, Richmond, Surrey TW9 1UR
  Tel: 01-940 4818
  National organisation with local branches offering advice and support for all forms of bereavement; may be able to put you in touch with other people who have experienced similar loss or may run groups for bereaved people in your area.

- **Divorce Conciliation and Advisory Service**
  38 Ebury Street, London SW1W 0LU
  Tel: 01-730 2422
  A London group affiliated to the National Family Conciliation Service (see below). Offers counselling help to couples considering divorce or separation, mediation to resolve disputes and conciliation over matters such as the care of children. Interested in the position of grandparents in such cases.

- **Families Need Fathers (a society for equal parental rights)**
  39 Cloonmore Avenue, Orpington, Kent BR6 9OE
  Organisation with 27 groups in England and Wales, as well as one in Scotland; publishes *Divorce and Your Child* and *Divorce – A Guide for Men* as well as a periodical journal *ACCESS*.
  FNF is concerned with the problems of both parents maintaining a relationship with a child if they have divorced or separated; holds regular advice sessions where individual problems about access or custody may be discussed.

- **Family Rights Group**
  6–9 Manor Gardens, Holloway Road, London N7 6LA
  Tel: 01-263 4016 or 263 9724.
  Advice only 01-272 7308 9.30 – 12.30 Mon.Wed. Fri.
  Organisation working to improve the law and encourage good practice concerning children *in care*; will give legal advice or put you in touch with a local specialist solicitor. They publish a number of booklets for families with children in care, including *Child Protection Procedures – A Guide For Families*.

- **FIRM – The Forum for Initiatives in Reparation and Mediation**
  19 London End, Beaconsfield, Buckinghamshire HP9 2HN
  A network of projects, organisations and individuals interested in helping people resolve conflicts; provides an advice and information service and runs training workshops; publishes a newsheet and a quarterly journal, *Mediation*. Contact them for details of any scheme in your area that might help you resolve serious difficulties within your family.

- **Gingerbread for lone parents and children**
  35 Wellington Street, London WC2E 7BN
  Tel: 01-240 0953
  Organisation with several local groups which arrange events and services for one-parent families: a wide range of publications, including a quarterly magazine *Ginger*.

- **Harmony**
  22 St Mary's Road, Meare, Glastonbury, Somerset BA6 9SP
  Group of families with children from different ethnic backgrounds, aiming to foster good relations and equality.

- **International Social Services**
  Cranmer House, 39 Brixton Road, London SW9 6DD
  Tel: 01-735 8941
  Counselling agency with contacts in many countries, which can find out details about the welfare of abducted children.

- **Interights**
  Kingsway Chambers, 46 Kingsway, London WC2B 6EN
  Tel: 01-242 5581
  Offers free legal advice and assistance to people bringing cases before international tribunals, such as the Court of Human Rights.

- **The National Association for Young People in Care**
  and **Black and in Care**
  20 Compton Terrace, London N1 2UN
  Groups of young people in the care of local authorities. An older grandchild may benefit from such a group. (See also, A Voice for the Child in Care.)

- **The National Family Conciliation Service**
  34 Milton Road, Swindon, Wiltshire
  Tel: 0793 618486
  About 50 local groups are affiliated to this service offering a number of services to couples (married or otherwise) to help them reach an amicable parting. When there are young children involved, the service will help people reach the best possible arrangements for the children. This service is not free but people may be helped if they are in financial difficulty. The Divorce Conciliation and Advisory Service is the London group of this service.

- **National Foster Care Association**
  Francis House, Francis Street, London SW1P 1DE
  Tel: 01-828 6266
  Association of foster parents and those involved in helping families who foster children; offers advice and information and publishes useful booklets, such as *The Role of the Natural Parents in Foster Care*.

- **NORCAP (The National Organisation for Counselling of Adoptees and Parents)**
  3 New High Street, Headington, Oxford OX3 5AJ
  Tel: 0865 750554
  An organisation offering help to adopted adults in the search for their birth or natural parents.

- **One Parent Families**
  255 Kentish Town Road, London NW5 2LX
  Tel: 01-267 1361
  An organisation for single parent families, which could be grandparents looking after grandchildren. A team of specialist social workers give individual advice; a wide range of useful publications.

- **PAIN (Parents Against Injustice for Children)**
  Conifers, 2 Pledgdon Green, Nr Henham, Bishops Stortford, Hertfordshire CM22 6BN
  Organisation concerned with children *taken into care*, campaigns for changes in the law and better practice by social services departments.

- **Parents Aid**
  66 Chippingfield, Harlow, Essex CM17 0DJ
  Tel: 0279 446103 (daytime) or 413768 (evenings)
  Group of parents with children *in care* who give mutual support and advice. Groups in other areas with a list of local contacts throughout the country; publish a newsletter and a *Guide for Parents with Children in Care* (price £1, available from the address above).

- **The Post-Adoption Centre**
  Interchange Building, 15 Wilkin Street, London NW5 3NG
  Tel: 01-284 0555
  Organisation offering couselling to any of the participants in an adoption; information and couselling help to all members of the birth or adoptive family, including grandparents.

- **Relate – National Marriage Guidance**
  Herbert Gray College, Little Church Street, Rugby CV21 3AP
  Tel: 0788 73241
  Previously known as the National Marriage Guidance Council. Local groups offering a free service to couples seeking advice and help with problems in their relationship. Often waiting lists. Some groups offer advice to other family members, such as grandparents. Address of your local group in the telephone book, perhaps under the former name. About eight per cent of couples seeking help from Relate are older people considering divorce or separation, or who have marriage problems.

- **Salvation Army Social Services Investigations Department**
  105–109 Judd Street, London WC1H 9TS
  Tel: 01-387 2772
  Attempts to trace and re-unite relatives who have drifted apart over the years, but only with the consent of the 'missing' person. Cannot undertake the tracing of children under 17.

- **Stepfamily (The National Stepfamily Association)**
  162 Tennison Road, Cambridge CB1 2DP
  Tel: 0223 460313
  Voluntary organisation for stepfamilies; publishes *One Step at a Time: Grandparents and Step-grandparents* (Erica De 'Ath and Linda Parry-Jones) price 40 pence. Local groups, a quarterly newletter and a telephone counselling service (Tel: 0223 460313) for all members of step-families. They have a national list of specialist Family Therapists for long-term help and counselling. Annual subscription £10.

- **A Voice for the Child in Care**
  60 Carysfort Road, London N8
  Group for young people who need someone to talk to about being in care.

BIBLIOGRAPHY

Bengtson, L. and Robertson, J.F. (1985), *Grandparenthood*, Sage Publications, Beverly Hills.

Bennett, T. (1988), *Guide For Families with Children in Care (or on a register): 101 Questions and Answers*, Parents Aid, Harlow. (Also available in Urdu, Punjabi, Hindi and Gujerati).

Brubaker, T.H. (1985), *Later Life Families*, Sage Publications, Beverly Hills.

Cox, K. and Desforges, M. (1987), *Children and Divorce – A Guide for Adults*, National Stepfamily Association, Cambridge.

Crawford, M. (1981), 'Not disengaged: grandparents in literature and reality', *Sociological Review 29*, 499–519.

Cunningham-Burley, S. (1984), 'On Telling the News', *International Journal of Sociology and Social Policy* 4, 4, 52–69.

Cunningham-Burley, S. (1985), 'Constructing Grandparenthood: anticipating appropriate action', *Sociology* 19, 3, 421–436.

Cunningham-Burley, S. (1986), 'Becoming a Grandparent', *Ageing and Society*, 6, 453–70.

De'Ath, E. and Parry-Jones, L. (1987), *One Step at a Time – Grandparents and Stepgrandparents*, National Stepfamily Association, Publication No 5, Cambridge.

DHSS (1985), *Social Work Decisions in Child Care: Recent Research Findings and Their Implications*, HMSO.

Family Rights Group (1986), *Promoting Links: keeping children and families in touch*.

Franks, H. (1988), *Remarriage*, Bodley Head.

Guthrie, D. (1987), *Grandpa doesn't know it's me*, Human Sciences Press Inc. (72 Fifth Avenue, New York, 10011).

James, A and Wilson, K. (eds) (1989), *Social Work and Family Proceedings*, Routledge.

Kivnick, H. (1982), *The Meaning of Grandparenthood*, UMI Research Press, Ann Arbour, Michigan.

La Fontaine, S. (1988), *Child Sexual Abuse, An ESRC Research Briefing*, Economic and Social Research Council, London.

Mitchell, A.K. (1982), *When Parents Split Up*, MacDonald, Edinburgh.

Mitchell, A. (1985), *Children in the Middle*, Tavistock Publications.

Mitchell, A. (1987), 'Children's experience of divorce', *Children and Society*, Vol.1, No.2, pp. 136–147.

National Association of Stepfamilies (1985), *The Step-parents' Handbook*, Hodder.

Packman, J., Randall, J. and Jacques, N. (1986), *Who Needs Care? Social Work Decisions About Children*, Blackwell.

Parkinson, W. (1988), *Separation, Divorce and Families*, Macmillan Education with British Association of Social Workers.

Pearce, N. (1986), *Wardship: The Law and Practice*, Fourmat.

Rowe, J. et. al. (1984), *Long Term Foster Care*, Batsford/BAAF.

Ryan, M. (1985), *A Guide to Care and Related Proceedings*, Family Rights Group.

Sawbridge, P. (1988), 'Adopting to a New Act', *Community Care*, pp. 25–26, 19 May.

Thompson, H. (1988), 'Divorce – The Split Sixties', Saga Magazine.

Tinsley, B.J. and Parker, R.D. (1987), 'Grandparents as interactive and social support for families with young infants' *International Journal of Ageing and Human Development*, Vol. 25, 4, 259–277.

Winn, D. (1986), *Men on Divorce*, Piatkus.

About Age Concern

Age Concern England, the publishers of this book as well as a wide range of others, provides training, information and research for use by retired people and those who work with them. It is a registered charity dependant on public support for the continuation of its work.

The three other national Age Concern Organisations – Scotland, Wales and Northern Ireland together with Age Concern England – form a network of over 1,300 independent local UK groups serving the needs of elderly people, assisted by well over 124,000 volunteers. The wide range of services provided includes advice and information, day care, visiting services, voluntary transport schemes, clubs and specialist services for physically and mentally frail elderly people.

Age Concern England
Bernard Sunley House
60 Pitcairn Road
Mitcham
Surrey CR4 3LL
Tel: 01-640 5431

Age Concern Scotland
54a Fountainbridge
Edinburgh EH3 9PT
Tel: 031-228 5656

Age Concern Wales
1 Park Grove
Cardiff
South Glamorgan
CF1 3BJ
Tel: 02222 371566/371821

Age Concern Northern Ireland
128 Great Victoria Street
Belfast BT7 1NR
Tel: 0232 245729

Other Publications from Age Concern

All these titles are available, post-free, from The Marketing Department, Age Concern England, 60 Pitcairn Road, Mitcham, Surrey CR4 3LL. Cheques or postal orders should be made payable to Age Concern England.

Your Rights 1989/90 by Sally West £1.50

A highly acclaimed annual guide to the State benefits available to elderly people.

Your Taxes and Savings 1989/90 £2.70

An invaluable guide to the complexities of the tax system as it affects those over retirement age and of the investment and savings opportunities available to them.

Using Your Home as Capital by Cecil Hinton £1.95

A best selling book for homeowners which gives a detailed explanation of how to capitalise on the value of your home.

Housing Options for Older People by David Bookbinder £2.50

This book looks at the various options open to homeowners or tenants, including special housing. Gives advice on sources of financial help for improvements and repairs.

The Foot Care Book by Judith Kemp £2.95

A self-help guide for elderly people on routine footcare, this book includes an A–Z of ailments, information on adapting and choosing shoes and a guide to who's who in footcare.

Loneliness – How To Overcome It by Val Marriott and Terry Timblick £3.95

Contains advice and information on learning to cope with feelings of isolation and includes real-life letters on the subject to Val Marriott – well known 'agony aunt'. The addresses of self-help groups and organisations that can help are also included.

The Magic of Movement by Laura Mitchell £3.95

Another encouraging book by author and TV personality Laura Mitchell for those who are finding everyday activities getting more difficult. Contains gentle exercise to tone up the muscles, and ideas to make you feel more independent and to avoid boredom.